World of Introverts

Embracing Your Unique Personality Trait

Gil Earl-Jones
MP Publishing

Copyright

© 2018 by Gil Earl-Jones

All rights reserved. This book or any portion thereof may not be reproduced or used in any manner whatsoever without the express written permission of the publisher except for the use of brief quotations in a book review.

Table of Content

CHAPTER I 6

BEHAVIORS AND PERSONALITIES: WHEN AND HOW ACQUIRED AND LEARNED 6

    NATURE V. NURTURE 9

    HUMAN'S EMOTIONAL DYNAMISM 10

CHAPTER II 14

WHO IS AN INTROVERT? 14

    AN INTROVERT BREATHES INTROSPECTION. 15

    FOR AN INTROVERT, SENSE OF SOLITUDE IS TANTAMOUNT TO COMPLETE AND TRUE PEACE. 17

    INTROVERTS CAN TALK BEFORE HUNDREDS OF PEOPLE WHEN REQUIRED. 18

    INTROVERTS ARE OFTEN MISUNDERSTOOD. 20

    1. Introverts are just a bunch of extremely shy people. 21

    2. Introverts see talking as a chore. 22

    3. Introverts evoke no emotion. 22

    4. Introverts get easily upset and nervous. 23

    5. Introverts always feel superior over others. 24

    6. Introverts do not perform well in school. 25

    7. Introverts are dull to be with. 27

    8. Introverts have depressive personalities. 27

9. Introverts are not considered as team players. 28
10. Introverts cannot assume leadership roles. 29

CHAPTER III 30

DIFFERENT TYPES OF INTROVERTS 30

1. THE SOCIAL 31
2. THE THINKING 31
3. THE ANXIOUS 32
4. THE RESTRAINED 33

CHAPTER IV 35

ACCEPTING YOUR INNER INTROVERT 35

1. DO PERIODIC EMOTIONAL ACCOUNTING 36
2. DO NOT ISOLATE YOURSELF TOO MUCH FROM THE CROWD 38
3. ON THE OTHER HAND, KEEP YOURSELF FROM TOXIC PEOPLE. 39
4. LEARN HOW AND WHEN TO SAY NO 40
5. MEDITATE OR DO YOGA. 41
6. CONSTANTLY IMPROVE YOURSELF. 42
7. DON'T MIND WHAT OTHER PEOPLE SAY ABOUT YOU. 42
8. DON'T BE TOO HARD ON YOURSELF. 43

CHAPTER V. 44

SUMMARY 44

CHAPTER I

Behaviors and Personalities: When and How Acquired and Learned

All of us are born into this world with a specific genetic makeup which we can literally call our own. From the time that we were conceived up to the moment we were born, we have since carried a specific physiological structure which gives us our identity and determines our behavior. This is something that is inherent in us.

The specific way that we talk, eat, sleep, or even how we react to different events in our lives are things only us can do. Our person is not something that can be transferred or relinquished. When one picks out certain traits they think are appropriate for them, they don't exactly reap a part of us that holds that same trait, but they instead try to copy and live by it. Our person, our possession.

Some are stout, some are skinny. Some have fair complexion while others have lighter skin. Some tend to feel ecstatic living all by their lonesome while others find peace when they are in a sea of people. Strange and complex, yes, but that's how humans are. Surely, we have our own characteristics which make us who we are. This is also why they say that each of us is unique, that there would always be something in us that would make us stand out from the crowd. No one has the exact counterpart, not one from anywhere in the world. Scientifically speaking, this is true. One might even say that each of us is patented, and we each possesses sole ownership over the same.

Imagine if all 7 billion people in the world share the exact same traits, behaviors, and beliefs. What if all of us are outgoing people? Will there be any need for alone time? Or personal space? Or Comfortable silences? The world will then become monotonous, only accommodating the same army of people, without diversity and texture. That's why when someone has a specific characteristic which is not necessarily what is possessed by most people, it is only fitting to be accepting of the same and not throw out biases and unfounded judgments.

As we grow, our whole being, specifically our behaviors, are being continuously shaped by many factors such as the environment that we live in and the people we interact with day in and day out. While it is true that we have unique traits built into our system, these also get influenced by some external factors that make us who and what we are.

The emotions that we feel are also largely affected by our physiological makeup as well as our exposure to different contributing factors. When we feel happy, the endorphins in our body must be working. When we want to cry, certain hormones in our body try to overpower other hormones to help us evoke such emotion. The external factors, however, also play an important role because without them, we would not have any reason to cry or feel happy. It could be a momentous event, your first love responding to your message, a stray dog drifting into your home, or a close family member getting assigned to a far off place. These emotions are what make human behavior interestingly dynamic and full of substance.

Nature v. Nurture

In pyschology, the debate between nature and nurture zeroes in on the percentage distribution of man's behavioral patterns that are inherited and those that are acquired or learned. By inherited we mean those passed on to the offspring through genes and acquired are those traits and attributes that one continually develop due to some external factors.

Nature concerns itself with the pre-determination of man's behavioral makeup affected mostly by genes. On the other hand, nurture takes its stand from the concept that man is continuously influenced by external factors he encounters immediately after birth. He then would have a multitude of experiences up his sleeve until he finds reason to use them, as well as the learnings and experience to certain variables which shape his way of thinking and belief system.

Man's physical attributes, the color of his eyes, the shape of his lips, the texture of his hair, his build, complexion, his blood type, including his susceptibility to certain diseases and his life expectancy have well been pre-determined even at the early stages of his development inside his mother's womb. And when he comes out into the world as a cute little baby, his whole character gets reconfigured to adapt to his environment. He then learns to have certain behaviors and start to lean to a certain behavioral sphere such as introversion or extroversion.

Human's Emotional Dynamism

When you hit your knee against the corner of a living room table or you accidentally dropped a 1000-page book on your right foot, a sudden internal desire to make revenge comes through. But since you have no one to target, as the pain that you have felt is mostly self-inflicted, you will just end up having pent-up anger. Or if you are angry enough and already in a state of obfuscation, you would probably take it upon yourself and punch something, maybe a wall or the very thing that caused you pain. Generally, this is how man reacts when faced with such situation. It is the normal reaction. When under pain, the first thing we want is relief. And most of the time, relief comes in different forms, depending on the circumstance and the degree of pain.

However, some people, especially those who carry a certain behavioral build, e.g. those who are a bit meek, coy, or shy tend to let it all pass and act as if nothing bad ever happened. Of course they would still feel the pain as the latter is purely physical and tangible. But the thing is, instead of dwelling on the pain, they would actually try to resist it altogether.

You see, we have here two extreme emotional spheres: one maximizes his emotions under pain, and the other subdues the whole string of stimuli and fight off the discomfort. Now we see why there are people who spend their time trying to exact revenge when faced with something uncomfortable while there are those who would rather keep track of what they were previously doing before the incident and try to move forward, allowing their tolerance for pain to kick in.

Each of us has our own way of reacting to things, depending on how we were raised or the environment we are exposed to. And through this process, some develop a certain characteristic which they take comfort in.

Some find happiness when they are with people. They tend to be more active and productive when they know that they are surrounded by those they trust. Even if the latter is not attendant, they would not find it hard to build relationships with other people, even with strangers. These people are hardwired to draw strength from the people around them. These people are commonly called as extroverts.

Others, on the other hand, would normally opt to be alone if the situation would allow them to. They usually feel a little off when they are surrounded by people, unlike extroverts who undoubtedly feel more confident and loved when in a similar situation. While these people can actually speak in front of people or be in their company if the situation calls for it, they, however, would choose to spend time alone. This type of people do not despise people. It is not at all the case. However, they feel more safe and secure when they are alone, not because feel superior than others but because they have a hard time getting their message across for fear of being misunderstood. This type of people are those we call as introverts.

The latter type proves to be fascinatingly interesting. This is because, naturally, man is a social being who yearns for recognition and care from others in order for them to survive. Humans are born into the world to co-exist with one another. That is just how it rolls. However, for introverts, the same might not always be the case. The interesting part about being an introvert, which will be one of the topics which will be discussed in this book, is how introverts actually feel more confident when they are all by themselves, away from the chaos that inclination to social relationships might bring.

In this self-help book, we will try to explain once and for all what being introverted is, how one with the said behavioral preference can embrace the same to live more harmoniously with the people around him. We will also try to bust certain misconceptions and myths about introverts. For one, many think that introverts are just extremely shy people, which in reality is disputable. By exploring the world of introverts, one would be able to identify his inner introvert and be able to handle such intricate personality.

Chapter II.

Who is an Introvert?

According to Merriam, an introvert is one whose personality is characterized by introversion or a reserved or shy person." Some define an introvert as someone who prefers solitary activities than interacting with large groups of people. The common definition of an introvert is that he is someone who likes to be alone most of the time, someone who would always have problems speaking to other people. He is someone who feels secure when inside his special and exclusive spot and feels deeply troubled when surrounded by people. Most of the time, this person gets the peace and quiet from staying inside his room or just by being secluded from the rest. However, his reality is not far removed from the one generally accepted by everyone. He just opts to find an alternative route in dealing with everyday things, mundane and serious alike.

To understand who an introvert is, it is essential to know who an extrovert is. Both personality types stand on a broad spectrum. What this means is that there's not one form of introversion or extroversion. Both come with different degrees. Likewise, there's one can be both an introvert and an extrovert at the same time, depending on the situation and attending circumstances.

An introverted person mostly carries such personality through a cycle of exposure to certain external elements. Although an introvert generally draws his energy and drive from his own internal world. A lot of introverted people acquire such personality because of the need to do so, especially when they are faced with constant stimulation from the outside world and the only way for them to cope is by erecting a wall only they could break or climb over. Some introverts have the trait inherent in them as part of their genetic makeup, in which case such personality stands no matter what the circumstance is.

An introvert breathes introspection.

If you are an introvert, then you love introspection. Introspection is when one finds time to examine and assess his mental and emotional processes. An introvert's personality is generally based on and grows through introspection. He is always self-aware and he often lets his mind wander through different concepts until he gathers information and ideas which allow him to create a world within, a place where he feels completely safe and secure. Again, this internal world is not entirely different from the external world, for the former still needs to get itself attached to the premises of the external, lest the person gets trapped in a world full of illusions. Although normally, the external world proves to be a breeding ground of notions and characters an introvert finds somewhat offensive, invasive, and compromising.

However, one problem an introvert has vis-a-vis his inclination towards introspection is that he tends to overthink even the simplest of things. Since he spends most of his time flexing his mental faculties, he sometimes gets submerged way too long and unnecessarily in a sea of thoughts and ideas, so much so that he starts to create mountains out of molehills.

For an introvert, sense of solitude is tantamount to complete and true peace.

While for most people, parties and big social events are a time for merry-making and recreation, for introverts, the same are concepts that bring chaos and disorder. For an extrovert, there's nothing like spending Friday nights out with friends and exchanging stories from the week's biz and buzz. Introverts find being alone as comforting. For them, there's some sense of peace through spending time alone. Solitude is what gives them time to analyze things that run through their mind and the same is what makes them able to keep track of their current state be it with regard to their work or life in general. But this is not so say that introverts despise going to parties. They also go to parties but they don't go there to meet new people for they are already content with being with those whom they are already familiar with. Normally, introverts feel alone in the middle of a crowd. They usually see themselves as outsiders when in gatherings or in activities attended by groups of people. However, when they see familiar faces, they then become at peace despite the busyness that engulfs the surroundings.

While most introverts find solitude as a good time for them to introspect, they don't, however, see downtime as something unproductive. They value the essence of resting and sitting idly by to rejuvenate and regain the energy that has been lost during the day. You are an introvert if you allot time for just sitting in a corner, staring blankly towards the ceiling, and trying to remove all the day's stresses. Introverts don't find shutting down after active work as a weakness or a waste of time. Instead, they see the same as a way to replenish. For introverts, even the simplest thing that involves the external world is something that needs much of their energy so the only way for them to carry on is if they spend some time per day alone and not thinking about anything. They think of the same as their way to cleanse and energize them for the days ahead.

Introverts can talk before hundreds of people when required.

If the situation requires it, introverts can turn into the best speakers or conversationalists. The only difference they have between those who are outwardly chatty is that introverts speak strategically—they only speak when needed. And often, when they do, you would be surprised by how sensibly they speak. They don't waste their time talking about things that don't actually make some sense.

You are truly an introvert when speaking in front of people doesn't bother you but getting to know each one of them is too much for you to handle. Introverts are actually good speakers, however, when the time comes that they need to speak to people on a personal level, they end up struggling. Get them to give speeches but never ask them to meet people individually because the same would just prove to be cumbersome. Again, introverts don't hate people. They just have a hard time dealing with situations where they need to reveal a part of themselves to people, which is why most of the time, other people see introverts as extremely quiet and reserved.

Small talks do not interest an introvert either. If anything, introverts see them as compromising situations where anxiety attacks are highly probable. So instead of striking up a conversation with random people, they just end up staying away to prevent any further awkwardness. This is also one of the reasons why introverts are seen as too stiff and serious. Saying hello to someone an introvert is not close with is a tedious task for him, even more so when he is made to crack jokes. The tendency is that introverts are often seen as intense and intimidating. But don't get introverts wrong. When you are able to really get to know one, you will see that introverts are actually extremely soft on the inside. One might even say that introverts are adorably warm and kind-hearted. Well, good luck with breaking through their metaphorical wall!

Introverts are often misunderstood.

Unlike extroverts whose actions are pretty much on the surface easy to decipher, introverts think differently and act in a very different manner. It is probably because they take some amount of time before they can warm up to people. So as a result, introverts are often seen as people who are hard to understand. But the thing here is understanding introverts require a bit of deep-learning, something that goes beyond the normal hi's and hello's. You are an introvert when you more often than not get misunderstood. Like when you do or say something and people get it as the total opposite.

However, there are a multitude of misconceptions about introverts that would actually turn out to be entirely the reverse depending on the reference frame. When you actually exert some effort trying to know an introvert, you will realize that what their acts or words sometimes mean different. Below are some of the misconceptions about introverts and what they actually mean through the eyes of an introvert.

1. Introverts are just a bunch of extremely shy people.

Well, the truth is that introverts can be the friendliest bunch of people when needed. You are an introvert when you can transform into a social beast when required. Even discussing a concept or selling an idea then become something that seems inherent in you. However, most of the time, introverts would opt to just zone out away from the crowd. But to get it straight, introverts are not necessarily shy people. There is a big difference between being shy and being an introvert. The two are completely different concepts.

2. Introverts see talking as a chore.

Not entirely true. Most of the time, Introverts just prefers to listen, analyze what is being said to them, and try to come up with a really good response rather than initiating the conversation and feeding the other end with information that does not carry much sense and truth. It's not like they do not like talking, it is just that they will leave most of it to you. But make no mistake, when you hit it off with them or when it comes to topics and things that they feel extremely passionate about, they would not for a second think of just being merely on the receiving end of the conversation. They will surely offer you deep and meaningful conversations. That is their magic.

3. Introverts evoke no emotion.

This is a misconception that should be busted altogether. Contrary to popular belief, introverts actually just share the same emotional wavelength as extroverts. They, too, can evoke all sorts of emotions as any other human being. The only possible difference is that what they feel does not necessarily translate to physical acts, gestures, or facial expressions, or those that can be easily noticed by other people. When you see an introvert standing in the corner, don't be quick to judge that that person is could be the most emotionless human being you have ever come to know. You will be surprised at how complex and intricate their emotions can be. Perhaps, their edge is that they just know how to handle them instead of blatantly bursting out of anger.

When a certain emotion strikes them, they sincerely feel such emotion but their introversion just comes into play that is why they usually would end up not showing the slightest hint of fear, or anger, or happiness on their faces. That being said, there are however other types of introverts who are able to do so since not all introverts share the same characteristics. What lays the common ground is what happens after the encounter, because that is when they start to analyze how they reacted during the whole time and feel a bit uncomfortable. This part is when they start to become invested in controlling their emotions. The more they engage in similar circumstances, the higher their wall gets.

4. Introverts get easily upset and nervous.
While it is true that introverts are less aggressive than extroverts and sometimes they are seen as soft-

hearted and shy, introverts are actually confident enough in their own skin that they don't mind being in compromising situations where others would normally feel giddy or nervous. They may look nervous sometimes especially when they are with strangers (with the exception of one type of introvert which we will discuss in detail in the next chapter), but it is actually easy for them to regain composure as soon as they realize that they can go back to the little world they have created for themselves. Again, it all boils down to how introverts can control their emotions and not get too soaked up. They may feel upset at certain things but they don't let the same stand in the way of their everyday dealings and work. Who does not get all upset and nervous, anyway? Introverts most certainly do but they have the ability to work it out to their advantage. Besides, introverts are known for being firm and not easily swayed by whatever is thrown at them.

5. Introverts always feel superior over others.

Well, to set the record straight, some people actually feel superior over other people but the same is not necessarily true because they are introverts or extroverts. It is just the way that it is. But generally, introverts are the exact opposite. You are an introvert when you recognize other people's wins including their strengths and abilities.

But while this may be true, you do not deliberately and unnecessarily dwell on meddling with other people's lives. When you feel strong and able, you do not try to measure other people's strength and ability to make you feel more superior. While there may be some bad sides to it, it is actually beneficial for introverts the fact that they often just focus on themselves rather than trying to gauge other people and measure their abilities. This does not make introverts selfish or self-serving. Not at all. If anything, they just act this way because surviving for them is not solely about competing with other people around their circle. This is also why introverts can co-exist with people from the outside while they are safe and sound in their own little corner.

6. Introverts do not perform well in school.

All because people think that going to school means putting one's people skills to good use, in which case introverts won't fare well because of their lack of said skills—another misconception all on its own. Truth is, there are quite a lot of introverts that perform well in school or in any other activities or organizations they belong. Having people skills might be a requirement especially when it comes to school and work but there are surely avenues where introverts can show their talents and skills and maximize them to their advantage.

Many think that introverts are underachievers because of the culture that we have wherein those who are outgoing, outspoken, and fierce are the ones who excel in life. Some would even say that fortune favors the bold.

However, it is not all the time that the same applies. Truth be told, there are thousands (or even millions) of people who have reserved personalities and they are successful in their respective fields, be it in the world of fashion, science, sports, entertainment, politics, health, and philosophy. Even more so when it comes to arts because introverted people have high inclination to anything that is artsy. Since introverts do not usually have some solid modes where they can express what they feel, they resort to other forms such as arts where they do not necessarily do the physical part of expressing themselves. And often they really turn out to be good at making artsy things whether through music, on canvas, or anything that calls for high creativity and imaginative thinking.

7. Introverts are dull to be with.

This deserves a resounding no. Introverts may take time before they reveal their true self to people but this does not mean that they will bore you out the whole time you are with them. In fact, when they begin warming up to people, they would then start telling you interesting stories that you would yearn for more. However hard other people try to make of introverts as boring people, the truth is that introverts sure know how to have fun. The way they celebrate fun times may not be as intense as others would usually do but it cannot be denied that introverts know when to have fun and actually make the most out of it when such times come by.

8. Introverts have depressive personalities.

Introverts are often depicted as people who wallow in depression and extreme melancholia. Since they would prefer being alone most of the time, other people assume that they live in a lonely world where the only people who understand them are themselves.

This is particularly true because the general notion is that when one is alone, he must be lonely. But in the case of introverts, this is not necessarily true. In fact, when introverts are alone, they feel most free. They feel genuine happiness when they are in their self-made world. Introverts do not see being alone as a sign of depression. They see it more as a form of independence, in which case they feel all the more confident and strong.

They actually know how to spot depression so they try to be careful when they analyze things. They maintain for themselves a certain level of attachment to thinking, because any harder they think than the acceptable limit, the same would then result in depression.

9. Introverts are not considered as team players.

It's a given that introverts will not fight to be heard as they are wired to stay silent and observant most of the time. However, this does not mean that introverts are not team players. Every team needs to have diversity in its membership in order for it to carry out its tasks and meet goals efficiently. If everyone were a bit on the loud and aggressive side, it will be chaotic. While it is true that introverts prefer to work alone, they would easily transform into team players when the need arises.

10. Introverts cannot assume leadership roles.

The total opposite is considered as true. There have been several studies that show that introverts are actually great at leading teams. This is because they do not see their coworkers as competitors hence they always consider how they can help them be at their best. Introverts can lead because they use their thinking skills more than their use their emotions. They do not decide on things without first analyzing the pros and cons that are involved.

Most importantly, introverts have big potential in leading teams because they possess a certain type of confidence that does not border on arrogance and cockiness. They know how to listen so they are able to identify the issues that their members have which makes them really good leaders.

CHAPTER III

Different Types of Introverts

As laid out in the earlier part of this self-help book, I have mentioned that there is no single type of introvert. The saying "different folks, different strokes" sure finds application here. Since introverts come from several backgrounds and a variety of external factors affect each one's level of introversion, confining this personality trait in one box and categorizing them under one umbrella is not the best way to understand fully the intricacy of introversion.

Several studies have been conducted to determine the different levels and types of introversion to better come up with a clear understanding of this trait and avoid misconceptions and preconceived notions. According to psychologist and academic Jonathan Creek, there are four kinds of introverts and each one possesses a distinct personality trait that is unique to them. Creek named his model STAR which stands for Social, Thinking, Anxious, and Restrained.

1. The Social

The social introvert does not mind being in small groups but if he has the opportunity, he will surely opt to spend time alone. A social introvert puts so much value on alone time that is why if he has the chance he would do his best to avoid engaging in deep conversations with large groups of people who are mostly strangers to him. Social introverts cannot be entirely tagged as the shy type because they do not have problems with being with other people in social circles, at least small groups of people. However, they would always prefer being alone as that would make them feel more peaceful and away from fears and anxieties. Does a social introvert suit your personality?

2. The Thinking

This type of introvert is neither shy nor particularly fine with joining small or large groups. These introverts do not really have an inkling to a certain type of preference. More often than not, the thinking introverts are seen as extremely reserved because they prefer to wander and get lost in their own thoughts. During the whole process, the thinking introverts get to put their creativity and imagination to good use, especially in a way that brings out interesting concepts and ideas and not vague abstracts, illusions which would just often result in neurosis. Are you a thinking introvert?

3. The Anxious

These are the introverts who always feel self-conscious whenever they are around people, especially strangers. These introverts somewhat closely resemble society's idea of a quiet individual. They are often socially awkward and whenever they are in large groups of people they would surely spend time calculating their steps and making sure that no one is judging them or they are not in any manner ruining their chance at establishing relationships with people. And if they in fact do, they would spend the rest of their time obsessing about how they ruined the occasion and what other people make of their behavior and overall personality trait.

Sadly, the anxious introverts get nervous around people, so much so that their only way to escape from the uncomfortable situation is if they find solitude someplace else. This trait of the anxious introvert can be attributed to lack of confidence. Anxious introverts are not particularly confident in their social skills that is why they find it hard to build relationships with other people. Do you see yourself as an anxious introvert?

4. The Restrained

The restrained introverts are not necessarily socially awkward, imaginative, or prefer to be with small groups or better all by their lonesome. These introverts' unique trait is that they move in their own phase, although most of the time they do it slowly. These introverts always make sure to pour some time thinking and analyzing their actions or words before they execute or say them (advantageous, mostly).

These introverts are those who usually think before they speak or those who spend some time the consequences of their actions before they carry out the same. Essentially, they are the cautious type of introverts. While their being slow can have some negative sides especially when it comes to fast-paced work environments, the good thing about being a restrained introvert is that you are sure that what you are doing or saying actually have undergone some sufficient processing that chances of ruining things is far removed from happening. Do you possess any of the traits of a restrained introvert?

While there are several types of introverts, it is interesting to note that there's not one single type that anyone who is generally introverted can be categorized under. A specific type of introvert would sometimes have some traits that are particularly observed on people who fall under a different type. This is completely normal. Besides, there is no one-size-fits-all category to define this personality trait.

CHAPTER IV

Accepting Your Inner Introvert

Now that you have understood how an introvert's mind works and probably at this point you have already determine what kind of introvert that you are, you are now more able to deal with your emotions better and establish relationships without hurting anyone or putting yourself in a very prejudicial situation.

Some introverts try hard to fight off their personality trait all because they entertain negative remarks coming from other people. Sometimes, the pressure to change really becomes burdensome and heavy because the people around them are too quick to judge. This is also why it is important for an introvert to surround themselves with people who truly understand and accept who they are because at the end of the day, they are just like any other human beings who carry unique traits which make them truly outstanding.

Being an introvert does not mean you have to conform to what is accepted by the society and try to fit in. You don't have to because you are born with unique traits that make you who you are, and that's something no one can ever discriminate against. The first thing that you need to do is accept your inner introvert, your personality trait. Embrace it. It sure is something that will make you a cut above the rest. Here are some tips you can consider to make introversion your friend.

1. Do periodic emotional accounting.

Being self-aware at times will help you identify negative triggers and allow you to maximize positive thoughts. You can do periodic emotional accounting to determine negative thoughts that shape your outlook. This will help you understand yourself better, how you respond to other people's actions, and how you can react differently if you find yourself struggling during those encounters.

Observe your thoughts and feelings. Try to make an inventory of the emotions you would usually have on a day-to-day basis. It can be just a mental list or if you have time, you can write them down. Make some observations. Do you often feel angry? Do usually get upset or nervous whenever you're around people? Do certain external processes make you feel uncomfortable? Through this process, your mind becomes aware of your inner self, the things that make you angry and those that calm your senses.

When you are able to identify from all the negative vibes come from, then you will be able to funnel down your energy on things that bring positivity to your life. Doing so will help you develop emotional stability and allow you to control your emotions whenever you are in situations that make you feel troublesome. Mind awareness in one important way for you to improve your EQ and make your life better than it already is.

2. Do not isolate yourself too much from the crowd.

It pays to build friendships with other people, especially those whom you think can help you develop your social skills. These should not be just shallow friendships but deep relationships that can stand the test of time.

As an introvert, you surely yearn for genuine care and affection and the only way for you to do this is if you go out and meet people. There will surely be a bunch of people who are waiting to know you are and make friends with you. Do not be scared. Those who reach out to you surely have something to teach you, be it about life, career, or self-improvement.

Do not hesitate to speak to them on a personal level. This way, you are not only creating for yourself a zone where you can feel loved and cared for but you also get to contribute to the community by sharing with its members the things that you know and are good at. You will never know what you will be able to discover about life and yourself so always put that smile on whenever you step out the door.

Sometimes, force yourself out of your comfort zone. This way, you would be able to explore things on your own, things that might turn out to be actually beneficial. This will help you lead a better life and make you feel a lot happier and more content.

3. On the other hand, keep yourself from toxic people.

The last thing that you need in life are people who drag you down because of the negativity that they bring or the bad influence that they have on you. These people would always stand in the way of you living a peaceful and harmonious life because they do not spend even the littlest bit of time trying to respect your interests and preferences.

These people are those who do not understand your being and would always try to tell you what to do and how to act, as if you do not have any capability to do it yourself. Most of the time, these are the ones who enjoy ruling over other people and imposing unreasonable things on the latter. If they are not relatives or family members, better to stay away from these people.

This tip actually applies to everyone. But it finds better application to introverts because many people think that introverts can be easily influenced and lorded over. Most people, especially extroverts think that introverts do not resist, that whatever the former tell to the latter, the latter would submit. This is all because people think that introverts do not have the ability to resist that they carry a go-with-the-flow attitude in life. At the early signs of toxicity from certain people around you, it is better to disengage to prevent any further damages.

4. Learn how and when to say no.

Don't let other people abuse your kindness by learning to say no. Whenever people ask you a favor or if they want you to do something for them, you have to analyze if it's the right thing to do, or if the same would not run counter to what you believe in. If it affects your sense of peace and makes a big impact on your personality and that it changes your being to something you are not comfortable in, then by all means say no.

Some people think that just because introverts don't often speak their minds and that they are not as aggressive and outspoken as extroverts, then they would not mind doing them a favor, even if it means that the introverts would be in a compromising situation.

Saying no is not bad. Not at all. And you don't have to feel guilty whenever you have to do the same. When one says no, that means he cannot or he doesn't have the capacity to do what is being sought to be done. This does not mean that the person asking should feel rejected. And you don't have to explain yourself either. All you have to do when turning down something is explain why you are not agreeing. That's it. A simple no sometimes makes everything easier and less complicated.

5. Meditate or do yoga.

If you are the anxious introvert, meditating would help you release the tension from your body. This will remove all the negative energy that is keeping you from enjoying a healthier and more productive life. Spend some time per day doing simple meditation and yoga. The results would surely be great. Meditating would help you improve your sense of focus and allow you to take control of your brain so that it would not get easily distracted. This will then allow you to think clearly and react properly when you are in any kind of situation. When you meditate, you allow your brain to relax and your body then follows suit. Meditation is good for the mind and the body so whenever you have time, be sure to go to a little corner of your house and try to meditate.

6. Constantly improve yourself.

Again, this applies to everyone. Always find time to do meaningful work which will give you a sense of satisfaction and fulfillment. Strive to add value to yourself whenever you have the opportunity to do so. Don't be afraid to take credit for the good work that you do be it in school, at home, or in the office.

7. Don't mind what other people say about you.

People always have something to say anyway. Learn how to shut your ears whenever you hear negative remarks whether it be directed towards you or to some other people. Whatever they say would not define who you are. Focus your time and energy on the people who truly love and care for you. These people genuinely care about what you feel and think so what they say about you is what truly matters not what other people try to make up about you.

8. Don't be too hard on yourself.

People make mistakes. We all do, extroverts and introverts alike. Don't be too hard on yourself. Whenever you commit a mistake, think of it as a learning experience more than a failure. No one will ever be perfect and human beings are bound to surely make mistakes at some point in their lives. These mistakes are what make us who we are. If anything, they actually help us improve ourselves. Don't blame yourself for every single mishap that happens around you. Embrace your flaws. These flaws make you unique and incomparable.

CHAPTER V.

Summary

Being an introvert is not a defect. It is a personality trait that makes anyone who carries it unique and outstanding. Introversion does not make someone any less of a person. In fact, it makes him totally different in a good way. Embracing your inner introvert, whether you are a social, thinking, anxious, or restrained introvert, entails some sense of understanding not just from the people around you but from yourself as well. As an introvert, don't be afraid to explore things and always aim to lead a meaningful and worthwhile life.

www.ingramcontent.com/pod-product-compliance
Lightning Source LLC
Chambersburg PA
CBHW030058230526
45471CB00003B/1155